DIVINE HEALTH AFFIRMATIONS AGAINST ARTHRITIS

.....A Therapy that Works....

BY
IHEKE WILLIAMS

COPYRIGHT © 2019, IHEKE WILLIAMS

Unless otherwise indicated, all scripture quotations are
taken from the King James Version of the Bible
A key for other Bible versions used

NKJV	New King James Version
AMP	The Amplified Bible
TANT	The New Amplified Bible
TLB -	The Living Bible
CEV -	Contemporary English Version
NASB	New American Standard Version
GW -	God's Word version
ESV -	English Standard Version
NET -	New English Translation
ISV -	International Standard Version
NIV -	New International Version
MSG -	The Message Translation

<u>DEDICATION</u>

This Book is dedicated to Almighty God and
to everyone in the world.

TABLE OF CONTENT

WHAT IS ARTHRITIS?

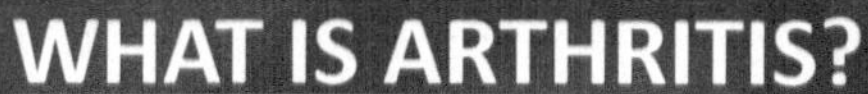

Arthritis is a term often used to mean any disorder that affects the joints. Symptoms generally include joint pain and stiffness. Other symptoms may include redness, warmth, swelling, and decreased range of motion of the affected joints.

Source: Wikipedia

<u>**WHAT IS GOD'S SOLUTION**</u>

"…By His wounds ye have
been healed.."
1 Peter 2:24

JESUS has already healed you
over 2000 years ago.

You are ACTIVE and STRONG
FOREVER because of the
wound Jesus suffered on the
cross for your sake.

You have no business with
arthritis or joint pains.

For the next 31 days, you will
affirm this blessing in your life
and you will live free from
Arthritis FOREVER!!

INSTRUCTION 1

That if thou shalt confess with thy mouth the Lord Jesus, and shalt believe in thine heart that God hath raised him from the dead, thou shalt be saved. – Romans 10:9

There has to be a connection with what you say and what you have in your heart. We believe with our heart, this is the reason you have to meditate on the gospel with your heart, believe it and then affirm it.

For the affirmations to be effective, you will have to meditate on the scripture (1Peter 2:24) for 5 minutes, in your heart, and then affirm it.

INSTRUCTION 2

"For our light affliction, which is but for a moment, worketh for us a far more exceeding and eternal weight of glory;

<u>While we look not at the things which are seen</u>, but at the things which are not seen: for the things which are seen are temporal; but the things which are not seen are eternal. –
2 Corinthians 4:17-18

Do not touch any part of your body that has been affected by this sickness for the duration of the affirmations. It affects the word in your heart when you keep recognizing the presence of a sickness.

Follow these instructions and your affirmations will be more effective.

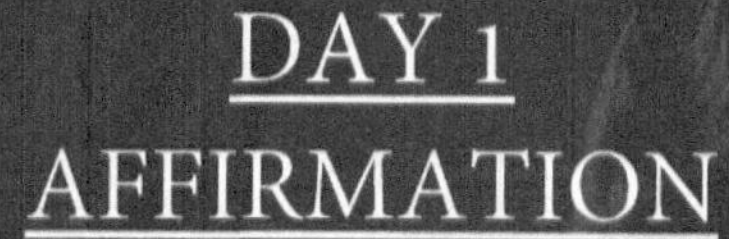

DAY 1
AFFIRMATION

Meditate on 1 Peter 2:24B in your heart for 5 minutes
"..By His stripes ye have been healed.."

Now affirm the Blessing

"I HAVE BEEN HEALED THEREFORE, I AFFIRM THAT I DO NOT HAVE ARTHRITIS!"

DAY 2
AFFIRMATION

Meditate on 1 Peter 2:24B in your heart for 5 minutes
"..By His stripes ye have been healed.."

Now affirm the Blessing

"I HAVE BEEN HEALED THEREFORE, I AFFIRM THAT MY BODY IS STRONG AND ACTIVE FOREVER!"

DAY 3
AFFIRMATION

Meditate on 1 Peter 2:24B in your heart for 5 minutes
"..By His stripes ye have been healed.."

Now affirm the Blessing

"I HAVE BEEN HEALED THEREFORE, I AFFIRM THAT I DO NOT HAVE ARTHRITIS!"

DAY 4
AFFIRMATION

Meditate on 1 Peter 2:24B in your heart for 5 minutes
"..By His stripes ye have been healed.."

Now affirm the Blessing

"I HAVE BEEN HEALED THEREFORE, I AFFIRM THAT MY BODY IS STRONG AND ACTIVE FOREVER!"

DAY 5
AFFIRMATION

Meditate on 1 Peter 2:24B in your heart for 5 minutes
"..By His stripes ye have been healed.."

Now affirm the Blessing

"I HAVE BEEN HEALED THEREFORE, I AFFIRM THAT I DO NOT HAVE ARTHRITIS!"

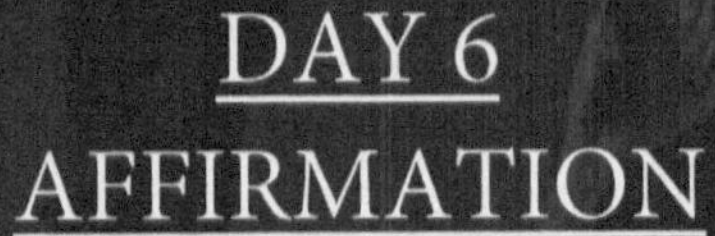

DAY 6
AFFIRMATION

Meditate on 1 Peter 2:24B in your heart for 5 minutes
"..By His stripes ye have been healed.."

Now affirm the Blessing

"I HAVE BEEN HEALED THEREFORE, I AFFIRM THAT MY BODY IS STRONG AND ACTIVE FOREVER!"

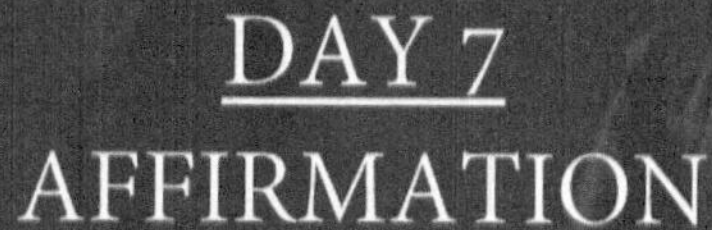

DAY 7
AFFIRMATION

Meditate on 1 Peter 2:24B in your heart for 5 minutes
"..By His stripes ye have been healed.."

Now affirm the Blessing

"I HAVE BEEN HEALED THEREFORE, I AFFIRM THAT I DO NOT HAVE ARTHRITIS!"

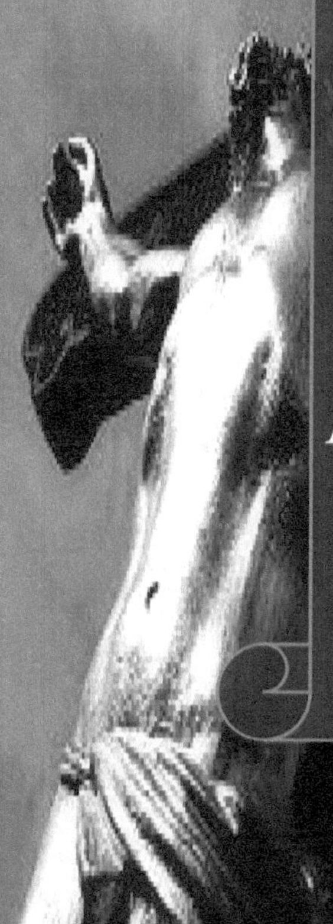

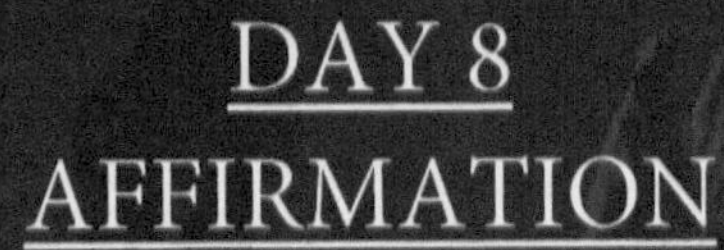

<u>DAY 8</u>
<u>AFFIRMATION</u>

Meditate on 1 Peter 2:24B in your
heart for 5 minutes
"..By His stripes ye have been
healed.."

Now affirm the Blessing

"I HAVE BEEN HEALED THEREFORE, I AFFIRM THAT I DO NOT HAVE ARTHRITIS!"

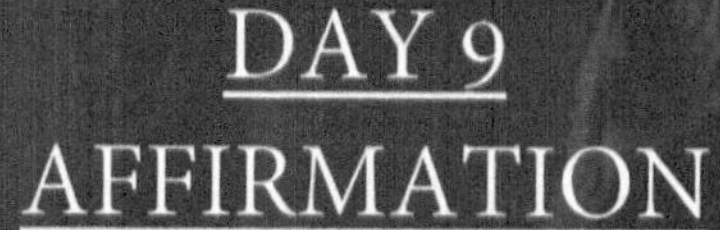

DAY 9
AFFIRMATION

Meditate on 1 Peter 2:24B in your heart for 5 minutes
"..By His stripes ye have been healed.."

Now affirm the Blessing

"I HAVE BEEN HEALED THEREFORE, I AFFIRM THAT MY BODY IS STRONG AND ACTIVE FOREVER!"

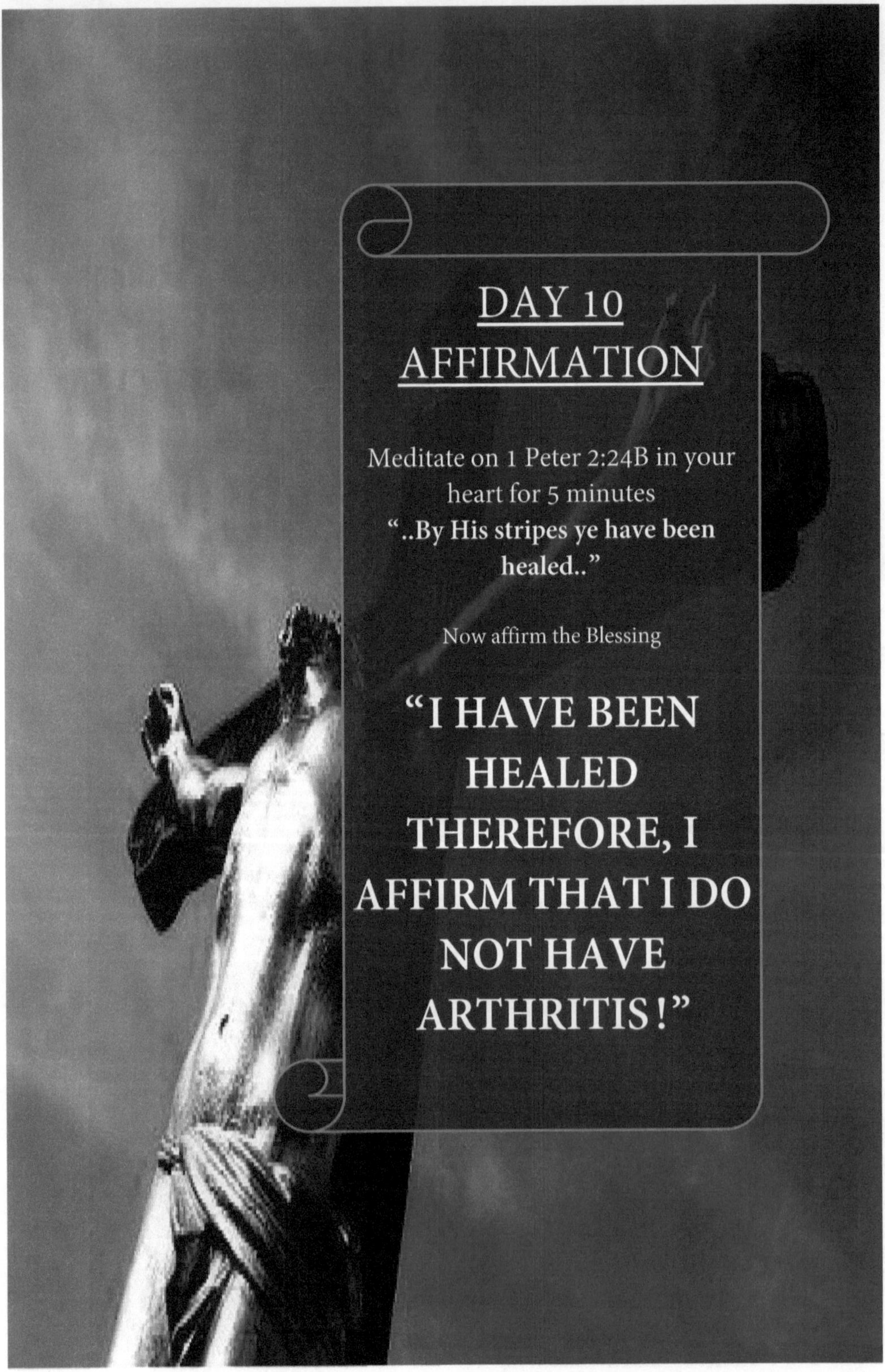

DAY 10
AFFIRMATION

Meditate on 1 Peter 2:24B in your heart for 5 minutes
"..By His stripes ye have been healed.."

Now affirm the Blessing

"I HAVE BEEN HEALED THEREFORE, I AFFIRM THAT I DO NOT HAVE ARTHRITIS!"

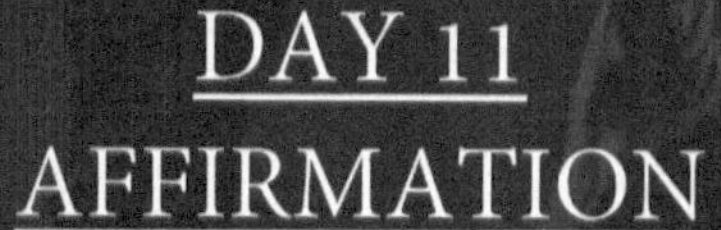

DAY 11
AFFIRMATION

Meditate on 1 Peter 2:24B in your heart for 5 minutes
"..By His stripes ye have been healed.."

Now affirm the Blessing

"I HAVE BEEN HEALED THEREFORE, I AFFIRM THAT MY BODY IS STRONG AND ACTIVE FOREVER!"

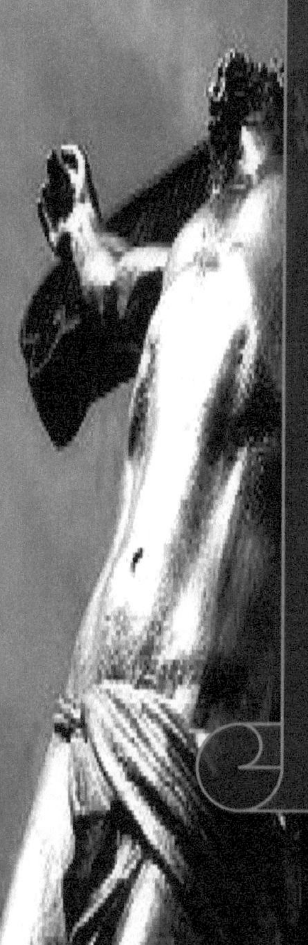

DAY 12
AFFIRMATION

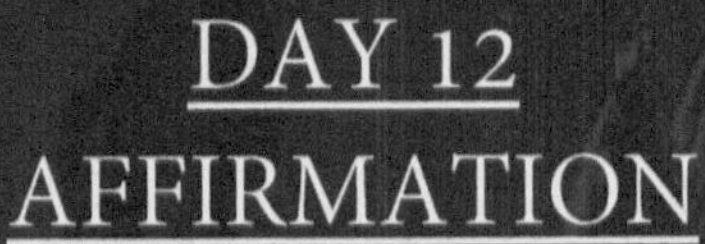

Meditate on 1 Peter 2:24B in your
heart for 5 minutes
"..By His stripes ye have been
healed.."

Now affirm the Blessing

"I HAVE BEEN HEALED THEREFORE, I AFFIRM THAT I DO NOT HAVE ARTHRITIS!"

DAY 13
AFFIRMATION

Meditate on 1 Peter 2:24B in your heart for 5 minutes
"..By His stripes ye have been healed.."

Now affirm the Blessing

"I HAVE BEEN HEALED THEREFORE, I AFFIRM THAT MY BODY IS STRONG AND ACTIVE FOREVER!"

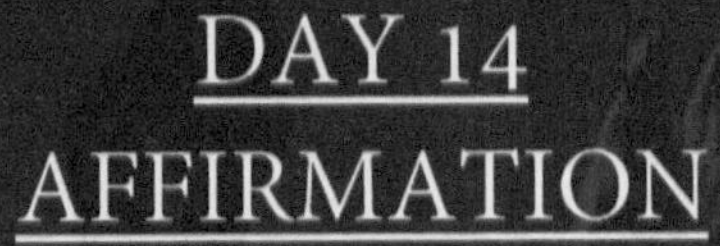

DAY 14
AFFIRMATION

Meditate on 1 Peter 2:24B in your heart for 5 minutes
"..By His stripes ye have been healed.."

Now affirm the Blessing

"I HAVE BEEN HEALED THEREFORE, I AFFIRM THAT I DO NOT HAVE ARTHRITIS!"

DAY 15
AFFIRMATION

Meditate on 1 Peter 2:24B in your heart for 5 minutes
"..By His stripes ye have been healed.."

Now affirm the Blessing

"I HAVE BEEN HEALED THEREFORE, I AFFIRM THAT MY BODY IS STRONG AND ACTIVE FOREVER!"

DAY 16
AFFIRMATION

Meditate on 1 Peter 2:24B in your heart for 5 minutes
"..By His stripes ye have been healed.."

Now affirm the Blessing

"I HAVE BEEN HEALED THEREFORE, I AFFIRM THAT I DO NOT HAVE ARTHRITIS!"

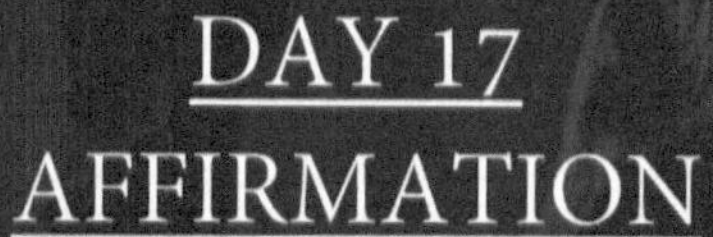

DAY 17
AFFIRMATION

Meditate on 1 Peter 2:24B in your
heart for 5 minutes
"..By His stripes ye have been
healed.."

Now affirm the Blessing

"I HAVE BEEN
HEALED
THEREFORE, I
AFFIRM THAT MY
BODY IS STRONG
AND ACTIVE
FOREVER!"

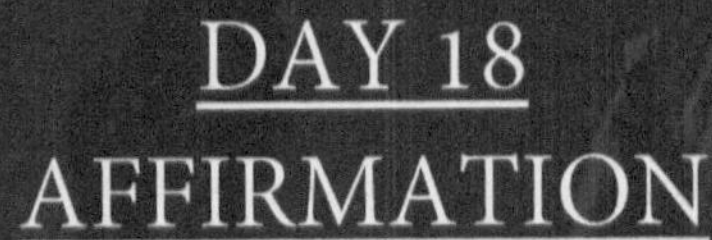

DAY 18
AFFIRMATION

Meditate on 1 Peter 2:24B in your heart for 5 minutes
"..By His stripes ye have been healed.."

Now affirm the Blessing

"I HAVE BEEN HEALED THEREFORE, I AFFIRM THAT I DO NOT HAVE ARTHRITIS!"

DAY 19
AFFIRMATION

Meditate on 1 Peter 2:24B in your heart for 5 minutes
"..By His stripes ye have been healed.."

Now affirm the Blessing

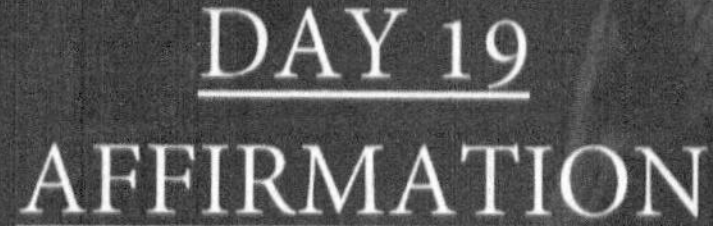

"I HAVE BEEN HEALED THEREFORE, I AFFIRM THAT MY BODY IS STRONG AND ACTIVE FOREVER!"

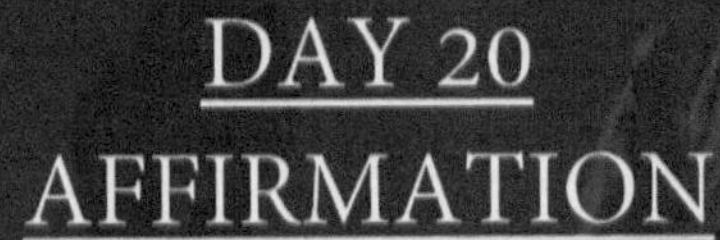

DAY 20
AFFIRMATION

Meditate on 1 Peter 2:24B in your heart for 5 minutes
"..By His stripes ye have been healed.."

Now affirm the Blessing

"I HAVE BEEN HEALED THEREFORE, I AFFIRM THAT I DO NOT HAVE ARTHRITIS!"

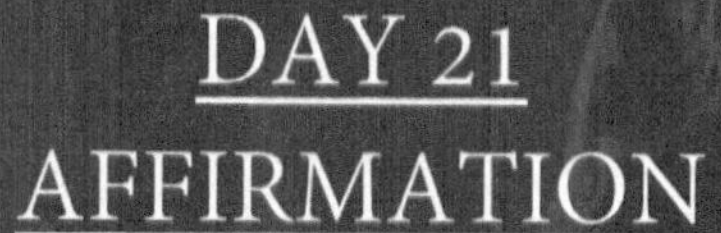

DAY 21
AFFIRMATION

Meditate on 1 Peter 2:24B in your heart for 5 minutes
"..By His stripes ye have been healed.."

Now affirm the Blessing

"I HAVE BEEN HEALED THEREFORE, I AFFIRM THAT MY BODY IS STRONG AND ACTIVE FOREVER!"

DAY 22
AFFIRMATION

Meditate on 1 Peter 2:24B in your
heart for 5 minutes
"..By His stripes ye have been
healed.."

Now affirm the Blessing

"I HAVE BEEN HEALED THEREFORE, I AFFIRM THAT MY BODY IS STRONG AND ACTIVE FOREVER!"

DAY 23
AFFIRMATION

Meditate on 1 Peter 2:24B in your heart for 5 minutes
"..By His stripes ye have been healed.."

Now affirm the Blessing

"I HAVE BEEN HEALED THEREFORE, I AFFIRM THAT I DO NOT HAVE ARTHRITIS!"

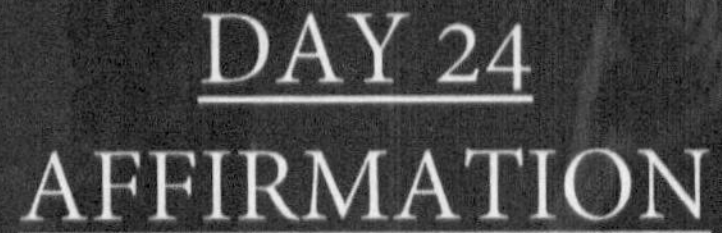

DAY 24
AFFIRMATION

Meditate on 1 Peter 2:24B in your
heart for 5 minutes
"..By His stripes ye have been
healed.."

Now affirm the Blessing

"I HAVE BEEN HEALED THEREFORE, I AFFIRM THAT MY BODY IS STRONG AND ACTIVE FOREVER!"

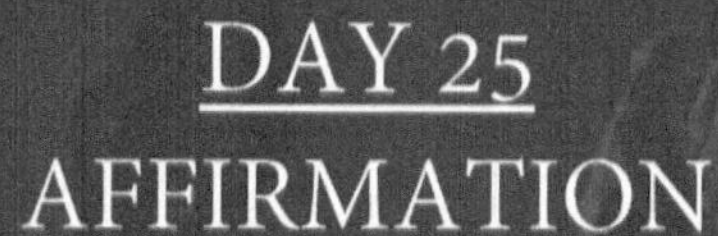

DAY 25
AFFIRMATION

Meditate on 1 Peter 2:24B in your
heart for 5 minutes
"..By His stripes ye have been
healed.."

Now affirm the Blessing

"I HAVE BEEN HEALED THEREFORE, I AFFIRM THAT I DO NOT HAVE ARTHRITIS!"

DAY 26
AFFIRMATION

Meditate on 1 Peter 2:24B in your
heart for 5 minutes
"..By His stripes ye have been
healed.."

Now affirm the Blessing

"I HAVE BEEN HEALED THEREFORE, I AFFIRM THAT MY BODY IS STRONG AND ACTIVE FOREVER!"

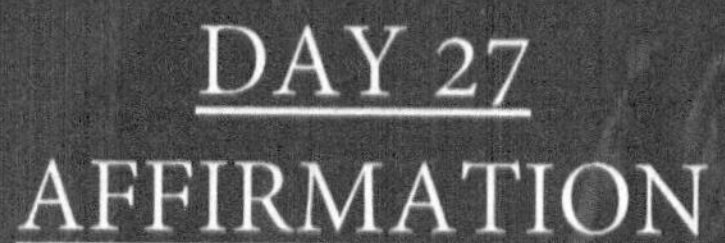

DAY 27
AFFIRMATION

Meditate on 1 Peter 2:24B in your
heart for 5 minutes
"..By His stripes ye have been
healed.."

Now affirm the Blessing

"I HAVE BEEN HEALED THEREFORE, I AFFIRM THAT I DO NOT HAVE ARTHRITIS!"

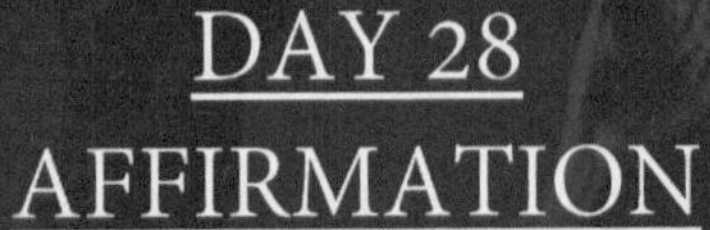

DAY 28
AFFIRMATION

Meditate on 1 Peter 2:24B in your heart for 5 minutes
"..By His stripes ye have been healed.."

Now affirm the Blessing

"I HAVE BEEN HEALED THEREFORE, I AFFIRM THAT MY BODY IS STRONG AND ACTIVE FOREVER!"

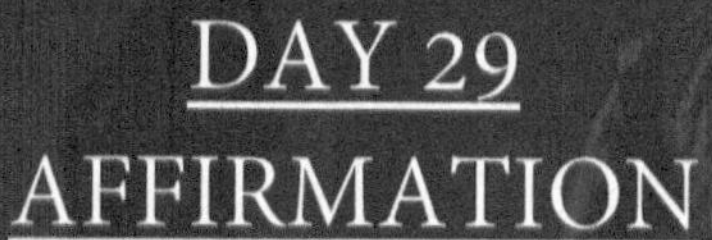

DAY 29
AFFIRMATION

Meditate on 1 Peter 2:24B in your heart for 5 minutes
"..By His stripes ye have been healed.."

Now affirm the Blessing

"I HAVE BEEN HEALED THEREFORE, I AFFIRM THAT I DO NOT HAVE ARTHRITIS!"

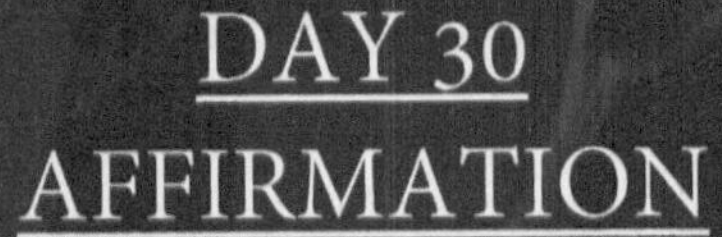

DAY 30
AFFIRMATION

Meditate on 1 Peter 2:24B in your heart for 5 minutes
"..By His stripes ye have been healed.."

Now affirm the Blessing

"I HAVE BEEN HEALED THEREFORE, I AFFIRM THAT MY BODY IS STRONG AND ACTIVE FOREVER!"

DAY 31
AFFIRMATION

Meditate on 1 Peter 2:24B in your
heart for 5 minutes
"..By His stripes ye have been
healed.."

Now affirm the Blessing

"I HAVE BEEN HEALED THEREFORE, I AFFIRM THAT MY BODY IS STRONG AND ACTIVE FOREVER!"

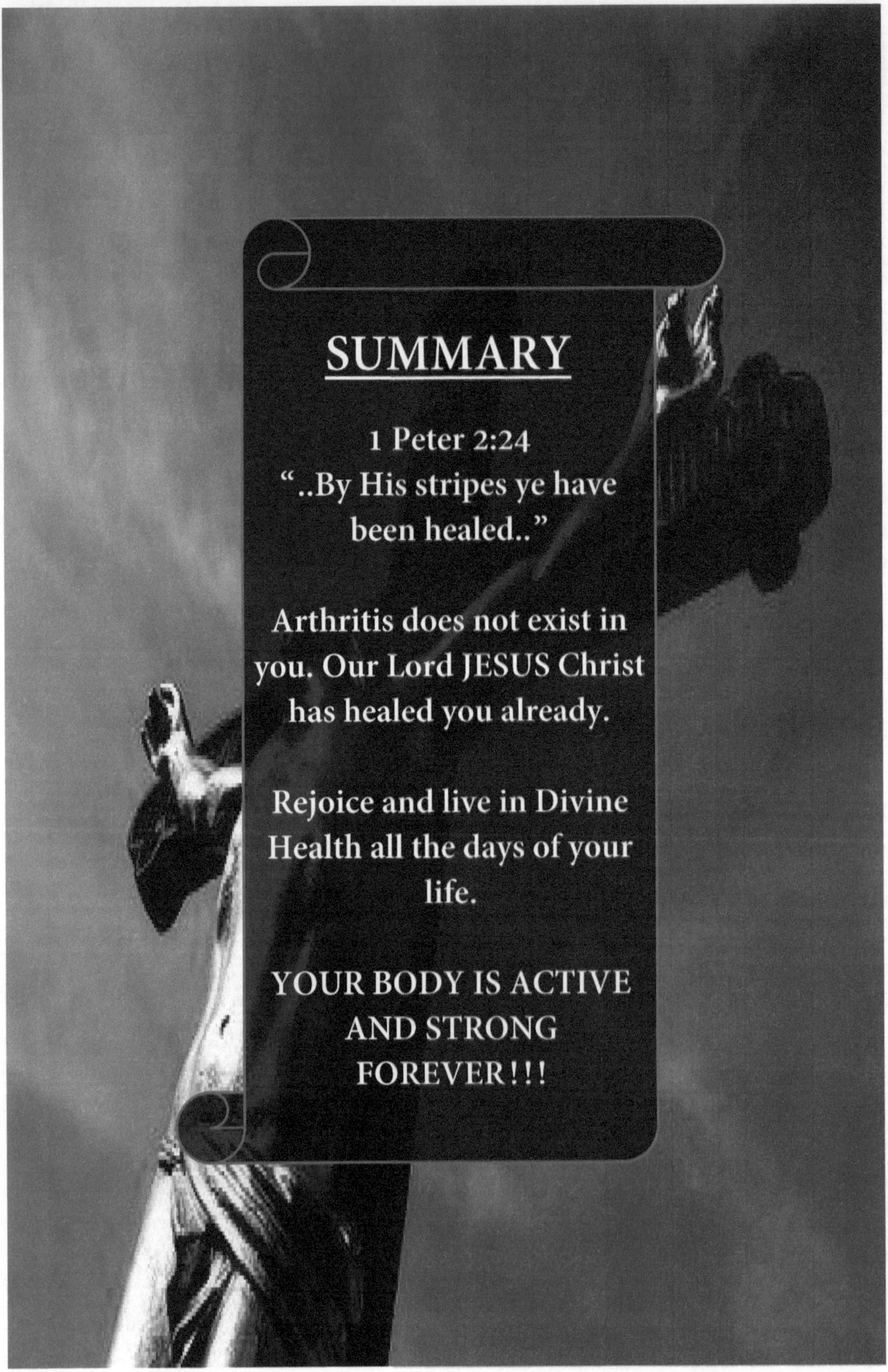

SUMMARY

1 Peter 2:24
"..By His stripes ye have been healed.."

Arthritis does not exist in you. Our Lord JESUS Christ has healed you already.

Rejoice and live in Divine Health all the days of your life.

YOUR BODY IS ACTIVE AND STRONG FOREVER!!!

<u>PRAYER FOR SALVATION</u>

We believe that you have been blessed and that you want to receive eternal life that God has made available to everyone who believes in his love and his grace which He expressed lavishly through His Son Jesus Christ.

"For God so loved the world, that He gave his only begotten Son, that whosoever <u>believeth</u> in him should not perish, but <u>have everlasting life</u>."
- John 3:16

Say this prayer to God and believe it with your heart

"Father, I believe that you gave me your only Son to die for my sin. I believe you raised Him from the dead. I declare that your son, Jesus Christ is the Lord of my life. I receive eternal life and I receive the Holy Spirit. I am saved forever.in Jesus name. I am so Happy that today and forever, I am your child. Amen ".

Congratulations, you are now a child of God Halleluyah!! – John 1:12

Other Information

Please share your testimonies via the following handles;

ihekewilliams@gmail.com
+2348061530541

Other Books written by the author includes
Dad, Pray for your Daughter
Mum, Pray for your Daughter
Mum, pray for your Son
Don't stop the flow of the Blessing
Daddy's Prayers
Mummy's Prayers
Divine Health Affirmation Against Cancer
Divine Health Affirmations Against Migraine Headaches
Divine Health Affirmation Series

About the Author

Iheke Williams is a firm follower and disciple of the Lord Jesus Christ. He is a passionate minister of the grace of our Lord and savior Jesus Christ and has brought the reality of the divine life of Christ into the lives of so many.

Iheke Williams has a calling to communicate the gospel of Christ with simplicity and to show the world how to activate the eternal life of God that is in us already which includes Divine health, Divine righteousness, Divine security and Divine prosperity.

As you read this book and other books written by Iheke Williams you will literally begin to function and manifest the life of God that is already inside you to the glory of God the Father who is the author of all grace and mercy. Amen

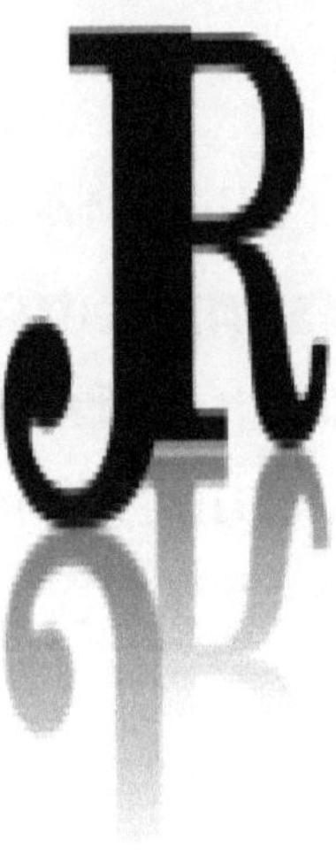